UNDERSTANDING MY SKIN

(THE DO'S AND DON'TS)

BOLUWATIFE MOBUSE

INTRODUCTION

So many people complain of their skins reacting to what they use on it. Why does this happen? Most people do not know. They don't find it easy to understand the reaction they have.

This book will make people understand their skin better. It will teach young and old how to care for their skin.

In this book, you will learn what to use for your skin. You will learn how to apply the techniques on your skin.

The skin; composed of water, protein, lipids, and minerals, is the biggest organ in the body. Your skin controls body temperature and defends your body from pathogens.

You should understand and care for the biggest organ in your body. What happens if you don't examine the biggest organ in your body?

An unexamined life is not worth living, said a famous philosopher.

How knowledgeable are you of the biggest organ in the body?

Before you can know and examine your skin, you should know your skin. What skin types do we have?

- ☐ **Normal skin**
- ☐ **Dry skin**
- ☐ **Oily skin**
- ☐ **Sensitive skin**
- ☐ **Combination skin (dry and oily skin)**

UNDERSTANDING MY SKIN
(THE DO'S AND DON'TS)

NORMAL SKIN

When we say normal skin, we mean a well-balanced skin. The skin may be greasy on the forehead, chin, and nose, but you find a balance in moisture, and in the overall sebum (the waxy, oily material that moisturizes and protects the skin). The skin is neither too oily nor under-dry.

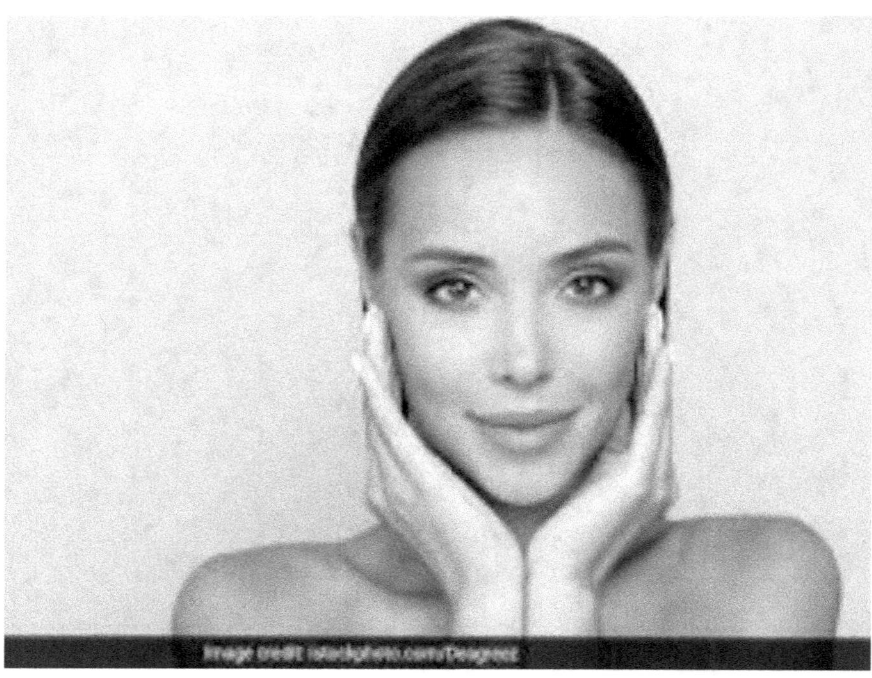

FIG 1: Natural skin

Symptoms of normal skin includes:
- seamless texture
- healthy radiance
- no oily or flaky patches, no obvious blemishes
- zero extreme sensitivity
- the equilibrium between sebum production and moisture content is well-balanced
- tiny pores
- a glowing complexion

In all this, we have to know how we can maintain a normal skin. So how can we maintain a normal skin?

I. Apply a broad-spectrum sunscreen (SPF 30 to SPF 50) to protect against UVA and UVB rays. Most of us are aware of how important sunscreen is for preventing sunburn and other harm during the summer, but we should use it as a year-round preventive health practice. No matter what the tone or color of your skin, always wear sunscreen. The usage of rice bran extract and jasmine to protect skin from the sun dates back to ancient Egypt. Many cosmetic and beauty products, including primers, foundations, serums, and creams, now contain water-resistant sunscreens.

It reduces your skin cancer: The most prevalent cancer in the US is skin cancer. The Centers for Disease Control and Prevention (CDC) report that in 2013, 71,943 people had cutaneous melanomas identified, and 9,394 of these instances were fatal. You can lower myour risk of developing skin cancer by using sunscreen every day.

It protects your skin from UV radiation: Sunscreen prevents harmful rays, decreasing the risk of being sunburned.

It prevents photoaging of the skin: UV-induced skin damage results in photoaging. A thick, leathery appearance, discoloration, and a breakdown of collagen, which contributes to lines, sagging, and wrinkles, characterizes it. According to studies, people under the age of 55 who use sunscreen had a 24 percent lower risk of acquiring these aging symptoms.

It helps keep an even skin tone: Sunscreen protects against UV damage's discoloration and dark spots, assisting you in maintaining a smoother, more even skin tone.

I. Wear sunglasses and a hat to protect your eyes from the sun.

III. Stay hydrated: drink enough water each day to keep healthy organ function, give

nutrients to cells, keep joints lubricated, avoid infections, and regulate body

temperature.

IV. Avoid wearing makeup in bed, and wash your face every day.

V. Moisturize your skin after cleaning it, using a decent exfoliation.

VI. Cleanse and scrub your face with good products to remove oil and dirt, then moisturize with good products to lessen the possibility of excessive dryness.

Is it possible to had have a normal skin but now have a different skin type?

Yes, it is possible. That is why you must take care of your skin by feeding it with the right food. Yes, the skin has its food; from water to lotion, moisturizer, to exfoliating scrub, soap and SPF.

DRY SKIN

Are you prone to dry skin?

What Causes Dry Skin?

Insufficient moisture in the skin-it dries out and becomes dry.

It might itch or annoy you.

Since your health, age, and the underlying reason of your dry skin can affect your symptoms, dry skin can affect anybody differently.

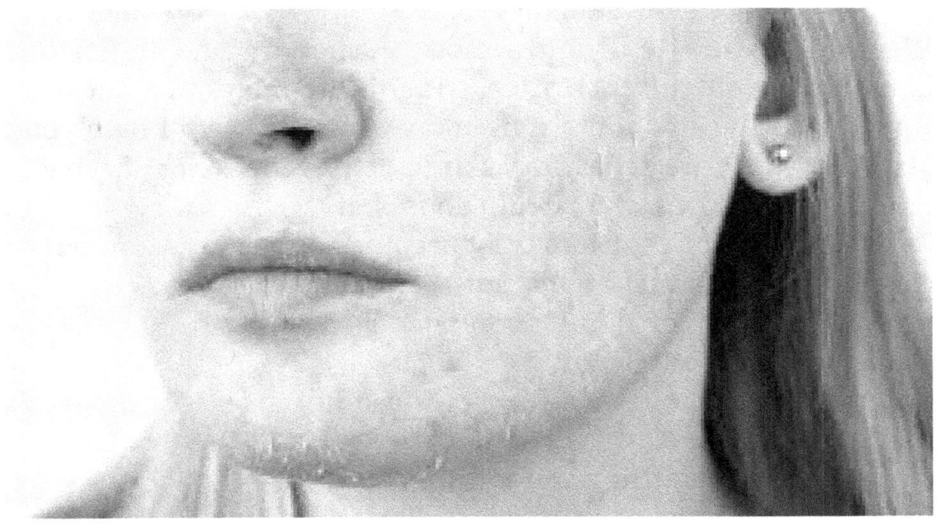

Fig 2: Dry Skin

If you have dry skin, you may experience these symptoms:

- Chipped skin (the cracks could be deep and bleed)
- Itching
- Blistered, flaked, or scaled
- Redness
- Rough-feeling skin that is gray or ashy
- Tight skin, following exposure to water (bathing, showering, or swimming).

Harsh soaps may contribute to dry skin since they suck away moisture from the skin's natural oils while removing them. So, one has to be careful while making the choice of suitable soap.

How can we relieve dry skin?
- Avoid using harsh soaps on your skin and rinse with warm water afterward.

Use a light soap, rinse with warm water, and take a warm bath instead of a hot one.
- After a shower, moisturize.

We should know applying a moisturizer with chemicals to a damaged region causes burning, stinging, itching, and redness. Applying a glycerin-containing moisturizer after will help your skin keep moisture, relieve dry skin, and prevent further dryness.
- Use gloves when doing housework

Take good care of your hands by keeping them away from harsh cleaners and dishwashing liquids that irritate the skin. When it's time to scrub, put on non-latex rubber gloves.
- Wash your bedding

Get rid of dust mites by washing your bedding at least once a week in water that is 130 degrees or hotter.
- Use hydrating hand sanitizer instead.

Alcohol-based hand sanitizers cause burning because they make the hands dry.

OILY SKIN

Oily skin occurs when the sebaceous glands make too much oil. Sebum is the waxy, oily substance that protects and hydrates the skin.

Sebum is vital for keeping the skin healthy. But too much sebum can lead to oily skin, clogged pores, and acne. Managing oily skin often requires a person making regular skin care a habit.

Face oiliness is a common problem.

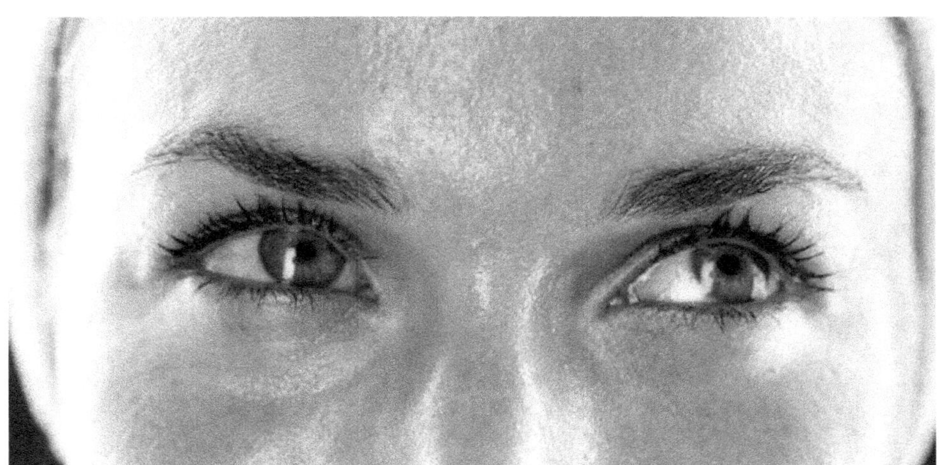

Fig 3: Oily Skin

Symptoms of oily skin include:

- a shiny or oily face and body
- large or noticeable pores thick or rough-looking skin
- occasional or chronic pimples
- blackheads and blocked pores

How we can reduce the symptoms of oily skin:

- Wash with warm water and natural soap (e.g., black soap)

    Stay away from soaps with harsh chemicals
    which can irritate or dry out the skin, making it
    respond by creating more sebum.

    There is no harm to the skin when you use a black
    soap containing natural ingredients.

- Avoid rough sponges, as added friction may stimulate the skin to make more oil.
- Choose the right face cleanser, which helps tackle oily skin.
- Pat the face dry

One should pat their skin dry with a soft towel when drying the face.

- Apply a moisturizer, which has 10% of aloe vera, aloe vera having a soothing effect makes it good for oily skin.

SENSITIVE SKIN

What is a sensitive skin?

The term refers to a skin that is prone to inflammation. People with sensitive skin may experience vehement reactions to chemicals and fragrances present in products.

What causes sensitive skin reactions? Causes of sensitive skin reactions include:

- skin disorders or allergic skin reactions such as eczema and rosacea.
- dry or injured skin that can no longer protect nerve fibers.

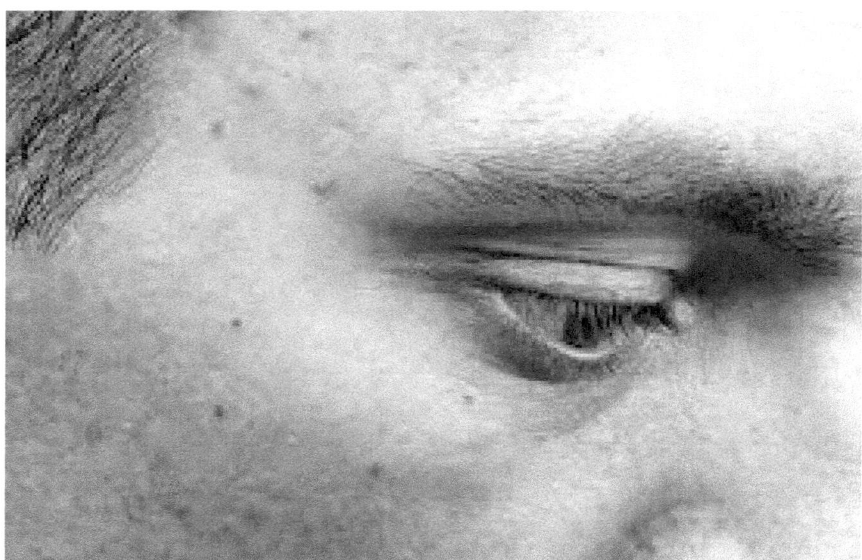

Fig 4: Sensitive skin

Symptoms of sensitive skin include:
- flaking
- redness
- rashes
- swelling
- scaling and roughness.

They can occur with sensations such as itching, burning, tightness, and prickling.

How to care for a sensitive skin:
- Cleansing. Sensitive skin reacts to various washing techniques differently from person to person. But most dermatologists concur that "deodorant" soap and soaps with strong fragrances should not be used on the face because they contain powerful detergents. Most liquid facial cleansers and soap-free cleansers like mild cleansing bars and sensitive skin bars have less of a chance of causing face skin irritation than soaps. The same is true for facial washcloths that are thrown away and washing lotions.
- Moisturizing. Skin can resist drying out and abrasion by

retaining moisture with the aid of moisturizing creams.
Avoid products containing:
Deodorant ingredients
Alcohol
Retinoids or alpha-hydroxy acids
- You should use a sunscreen with an SPF of 30 or higher. Titanium dioxide or zinc oxide should be the only active substances. Why? It's so you won't respond to allergy to these physical sunscreens. In contrast to chemical sunscreens, they reflect UV radiation from the sun rather than absorbing them.

COMBINATION SKIN (DRY AND OILY SKIN)

Combination skin comprises two different skin types, with the facial features like the cheeks having dry skin and others like the T-zone, the forehead, chin, and nose having oilier skin.

Combination skin symptoms include:
- oily T-zone.
- expanded T-zone pores, most likely with contaminants.
- dry cheeks are common.

How we can control combination skin:
- Keep the temperature of your products.

Store your products in the refrigerator, not the restroom.
- Use a quality cleanser.

In assisting the skin in maintaining the right amount of moisture, face cleansing routine is important. Skin that is dehydrated appears and feels old, wrinkly, and harsh.

By allowing enough water and product to be retained for skin hydration, cleansing aids in controlling the pH levels of the skin.

- Handle the cheeks and oily T-zone differently.

Twice a week, exfoliate. Excessive exfoliation can cause flaky, dry, spotty, and rough skin.

This signifies your skin's capacity to absorb or keep over-exfoliation has compromised

moisture. When this occurs, the results of your skincare and cosmetic regimen.

- Use SPF 30 to SPF 50

ACKNOWLEDGEMENT

Thanks to Almighty God and those who have help me greatly.

ABOUT THE AUTHOR

Boluwatife Mobuse

is a skincare specialist, who is interested in people finding their skin essence,irrespective of their skin tone.

Leave your comment

LEAVE YOUR COMMENT

CO